Cranial Relaxation Technique

A simple technique to calm the mind, nourish
the eyes and balance the nervous system.

Michael Hetherington

(L. Ac, Yoga Teacher)

Disclaimer

All material in this book is provided for your information only and may not be construed as medical advice or instruction. No action or inaction should be taken based solely on the contents of this information; instead, readers should consult appropriate health professionals on any matter relating to their health and well-being.

The information and opinions expressed here are believed to be accurate, based on the best judgment available to the authors, and readers who fail to consult with appropriate health authorities assume the risk of any injuries. The publisher is not responsible for errors or omissions.

About the Author

Michael Hetherington is a qualified acupuncturist, lecturer in Oriental medicine and yoga teacher based in Brisbane, Australia. He has a keen interest in mind-body medicine, yoga nidra and Buddhist meditation. Inspired by the teachings of many, he has learned that a light-hearted, joyful approach to life serves best.

www.michaelhetherington.com.au

Other Titles by Author:

The Art of Self Adjusting
Learn how to adjust the body for pain relief and better function

The Complete Book of Oriental Yoga
A journey into the 5 elements and yoga for the seasons

How to Do Restorative Yoga
Learn the art of a gentle yoga practice for deep relaxation

Chakra Balancing Made Simple and Easy
How to work with the Chakras for enhanced living

Increasing Internal Energy
Building energy from within to enhance daily life and strengthen our yoga practice

The Yin and Yang Lifestyle Guide
Yin and yang theory applied to modern living

Table of Contents

"Tension is who you think you should be, relaxation is who you are."

~ *Chinese Proverb*

Introduction

The aim of this book is to empower you, the reader, to be able to give powerful cranial rebalancing treatments to yourself and to others. This technique is very easy and effective, and anyone with the intention to help and heal can do it with little effort. What makes this technique so powerful and unique is that we work directly with the energetics of the brain, nervous system, and the acupuncture meridian system found in Chinese medicine.

After reading this book you will learn how to effectively practice this technique so as to gain the most benefit. Benefits include a rapid diffusion of any anxiety or stress, some pain relief from headaches, nourished eyes, and a general feeling of a calm and balanced nervous system.

You don't need to be a bodywork therapist or health professional to practice this technique—it is available to everyone, and everyone has the capacity to practice it. If you are a bodywork therapist or health practitioner, you may consider incorporating this technique into your healing practice if you come to find it to be suitable and effective.

At the beginning of this book we will go through each of the points, describing their anatomical location and the associated benefits. After that we will explore the 12-step sequence of hand positions so you can practice on yourself and on others.

I would recommend practicing this technique on yourself a few times before giving it to others so that you can experience its powerful effects personally. In this way you will be able to give it more effectively to others when the time comes.

The 12 Points

Before we get into the actual process of practicing the technique, we need to become more familiar with the anatomical locations of the 12 points we will be accessing on the head. Many of them are bilateral, meaning they are in the same location on both sides of the head. With each of the points, I have listed the meridian it is on (the energetic pathway according to traditional Chinese medicine) and the direct translation of the Chinese name to English to help give you an idea of the qualities of the point.

The 12 points are:

1. Gallbladder 14 (Yang Bright)

Anatomical location: on the forehead, in a slight depression about 1 thumb width above the eyebrow, and directly above the pupil of the eye if the gaze is fixed straight ahead.

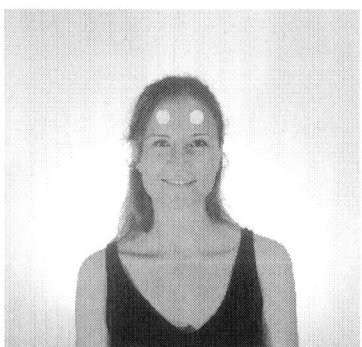

Actions: calms the mind, dispels heat and softens the eyes. Known for its ability to diffuse feelings of fear and stress.

2. Gallbladder 3 (Above the Arch)

Anatomical location: in the depression above the superior border of the zygomatic arch, just posterior to (behind) the temple region.

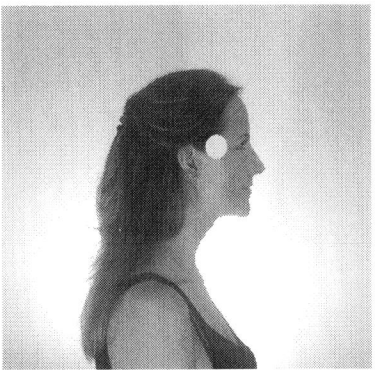

Actions: alleviates pain and tightness from the jaw and the temporomandibular joint. Clears heat and improves hearing.

3. Stomach 6 (Jaw Bone)

Anatomical location: at the prominence of the masseter muscle, one finger width anterosuperior to the tip of the angle of the mandible. Assist location by first clenching the teeth and feeling for the peak of the masseter muscle. Once located, release the jaw and hold both fingers on location.

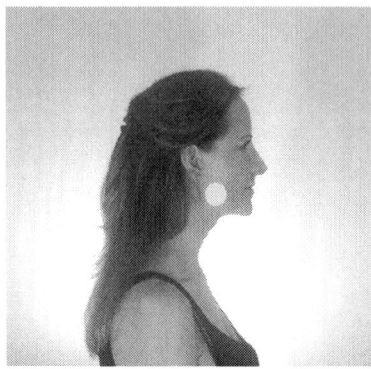

Action: alleviates pain and tightness of the jaw and temporomandibular joint. Calms the mind.

4. Gallbladder 15 (Head Governor of Tears)

Anatomical location: in a shallow depression on the hairline directly above the pupil of the eyes if the eyes are focused straight ahead.

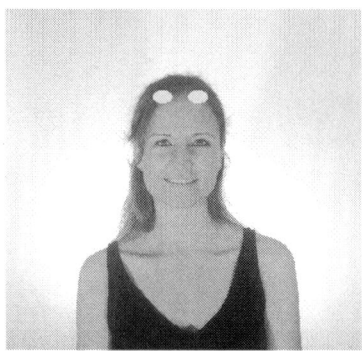

Action: calms the mind, relieves pain associated with headaches, reduces dizziness, and nourishes and moistens the eyes. This point is closely associated with the liver energy.

5. Gall Bladder 8 (Leading Valley)

Anatomical location: in a shallow depression about one finger width superior to (above) the apex (top) of the ear.

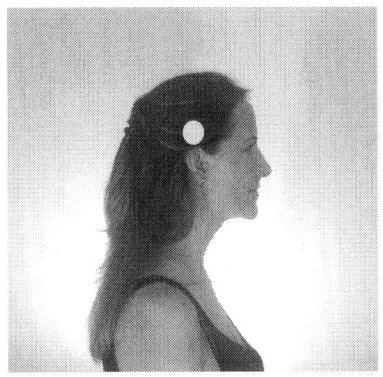 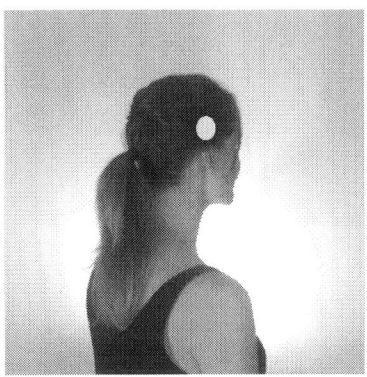

Actions: relieves pain associated with the ear or the temples. This point has a strong connection to spleen energy in Chinese medicine, as it helps to ground and calm people down quickly. This is one of the most powerful points on the head.

6. Gallbladder 17 (Upright Construction)

Anatomical location: in a flattish area of the parietal bone about 2 finger widths above Gallbladder 8.

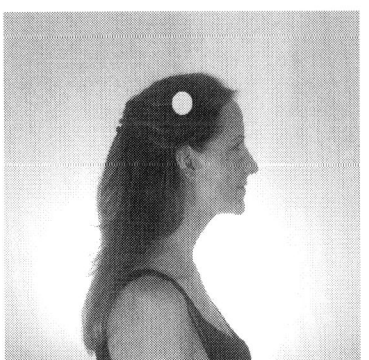 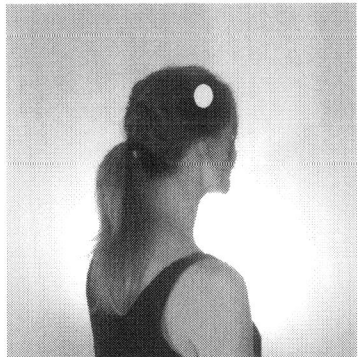

Actions: clears heat from the head to relieve pain. Nourishes the part of the brain that governs motor function (physical movement).

7. Du 20 (One Hundred Convergences)

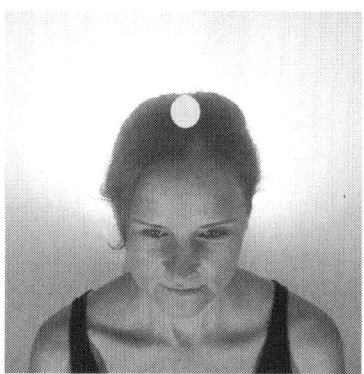

Anatomical location: at the vertex of the head about 5 finger widths posterior to the hairline. To aid location, find the midpoint of the line connecting the apex (top) of both ears.

Actions: a very important and dynamic point that helps to "lift" and balance all the yang energies of the body. It works to calm the mind, clears the head of heat and nourishes all the sense organs of the head. This is one of the most powerful points on the head and is associated with lifting the "heart" and spirit energy.

8. Du 19 (Behind the Crown)

Anatomical location: in a soft and slightly flat section of the skull where both parietal bones meet at the back and upper portion of the head. To aid location, it is about 3 finger widths above Du 17 (next point).

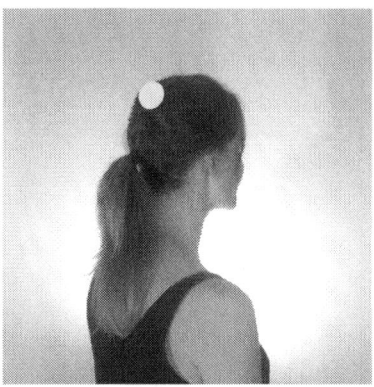

Actions: calms the mind, dispels heat and relieves headache pain, dizziness, or anxiety-related symptoms. It also has a nourishing effect for all the sense organs of the head.

9. Du 17 (Brain Door)

Anatomical location: in the slight depression directly superior to (above) the external occipital protuberance.

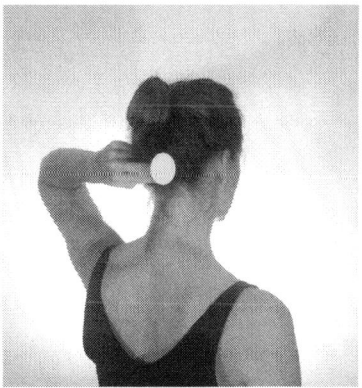

Actions: clears pain and heat associated with headaches, fevers, chills and helps relax any stiffness in the neck. It also nourishes sore, dry or irritated eyes and can help with any vision problems.

10. GB 19 (Brain Hollow)

Anatomical location: on the lateral side of the superior border of the external occipital protuberance. To aid location, locate the external occipital protuberance (ridge at the very back of the skull) and move about 2 finger widths to either side to find a flat area of the skull.

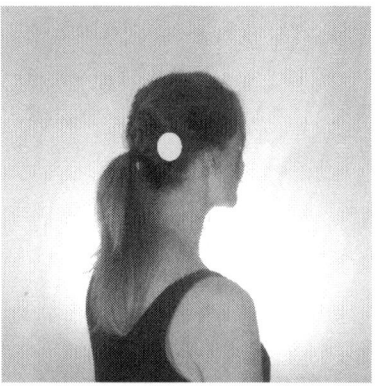

Actions: calms the mind and relaxes the back of the head and neck area. Helps to relieve pain and nourish the eyes.

11. GB 20 (Wind Pool)

Anatomical location: at the center of the large depression directly below the occipital bone, just within the hairline.

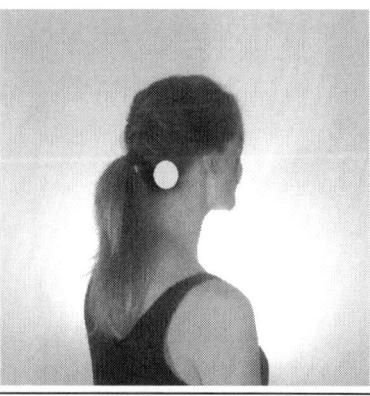

Actions: helps to relax the muscles of the neck and clears heat out of the head. Helps to support brain function and clear the sinuses.

12. Du 16 (Wind Mansion)

Anatomical location: directly below the occipital protuberance, in the depression that is made between the attachment points of the trapezius muscle. This point is slightly lower then point 9.

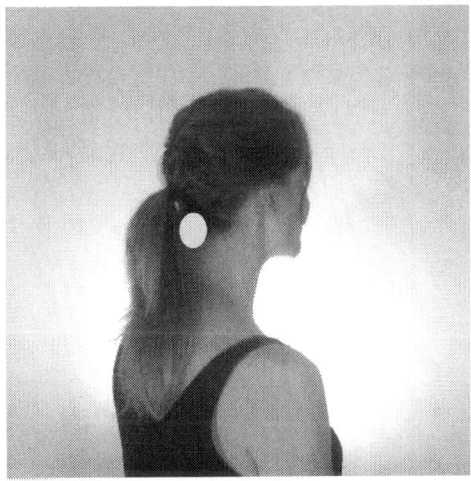

Actions: helps to regulate the nervous system. Calms the mind, relaxes the body and clears heat from the head.

Fundamentals of the Technique

There are 12 hand positions for each of the points explained in this book, and each point has its associated benefits as described in the previous chapter. For this technique we use the first and middle finger together on each of the points. We use the first and middle finger together because it has a balancing and neutralizing effect on the energetic system; more so than just using one finger.

The pressure of the fingers on the head is light and relaxed; we simply place the pads of the first and second fingers on the point. Allow the entire pads of these fingers to come into contact with the head in a relaxed and nurturing fashion. If done correctly you will quickly feel the warmth between the fingers and the head. You do not need to use strong pressure for this; it is not a massage nor is it some form of deep acupressure technique. It's a very gentle technique; the main benefit simply comes from the transfer of heat and electrical energy through the fingers. When we place our fingers on various parts of the skull, it naturally increases blood flow to these parts of the brain. It also helps to reorganize and rebalance the electrical activity of the brain, often balancing out the left and the right hemispheres.

The fundamentals to keep in mind when giving or receiving this treatment are:

1. A soft and relaxed touch of the first and middle finger on point location.

2. Make sure your body is in a position in which it is not straining. Rest the arms in between the points if they start to fatigue.

3. Use a natural, relaxed breath; no strain or effort required to alter breath.

4. Hold for at least 45 seconds to 1 minute, or 5 – 10 sets of breaths (breathing in and breathing out counts as 1 set) with the eyes closed. Be aware of changes in breath, or a feeling of a "fog lifting". Often the eyes become glazed and watery.

5. Have a drink of water after the practice.

6. This following may seem like common sense to many of us, but it is still worth mentioning. Please do not smoke, eat any sugared candy, or consume any fatty, oily foods soon after any treatment, as this tends to put the body under so much stress that it can render all the benefits from a treatment obsolete. Allow for at least 30 minutes after any treatment before engaging is such activities, or putting the body into a stressful environment. It is best to eat an apple or a piece of fruit, go for a gentle walk, get some fresh air, drink warm herbal tea and/or drink purified water after any treatment to help the body settle into its new state.

Self Treatment Technique

Ideally, set yourself up in a place where you won't be distracted or interrupted for at least 10 – 15 minutes. You can practice sitting in your favorite chair or sitting comfortably on the floor; just be sure to have your spine relatively straight, and your head and neck in a position in which they are not straining. For those who prefer to lie down, then lying flat on a carpeted floor or a bed, or lying on a massage table with your head supported slightly with a folded blanket are great options. You can even do this technique when you're lazing about in a bathtub or lying down by the side of a pool.

For each of these hand positions, just make sure you check your shoulders and allow them to relax by getting the sense that the hands are simply holding themselves in position without the need to stress or strain the shoulders. When you come to locate the points, close the eyes, find your breath and hold for at least 45 seconds to 1 minute (or 5 – 10 sets of breaths). Just let any thoughts or images that come up in the mind pass through. Don't give them any importance, just become the watcher and allow it all to flow through you without any impedance. Do not try to hold onto any of it or give it any importance by trying to place meaning upon it. The sense of space is more important to be aware of than the contents within the space. Simply allow the body to settle and relax into it. If your arms fatigue then simply rest them between the points.

Okay, let's go through the technique first as a self-treatment:

1. Place the fingers on the first point on the front of the forehead. Be sure to relax your shoulders, close your eyes and find your breath.

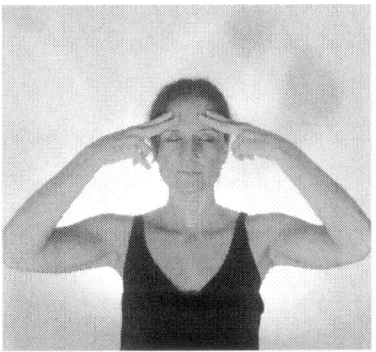

2. Place the fingers just behind the temples.

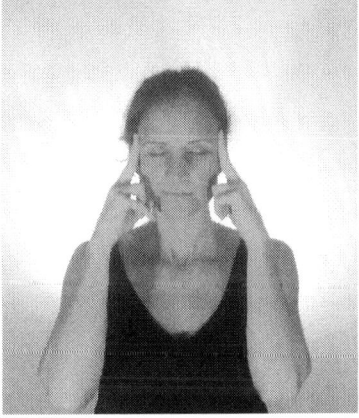

3. Place the fingers on either side of the jaw.

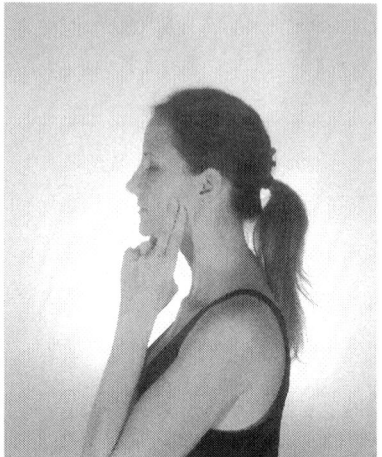

4. Place the fingers on the hairline directly above the eyes.

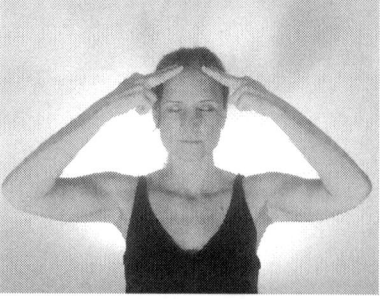

5. Place the fingers just above the tips of the ears.

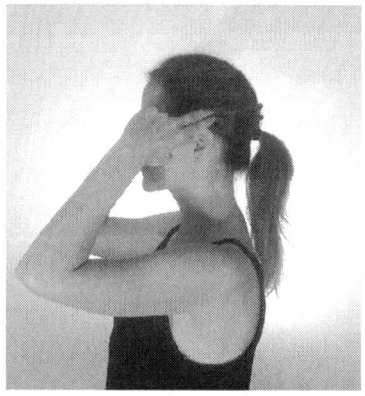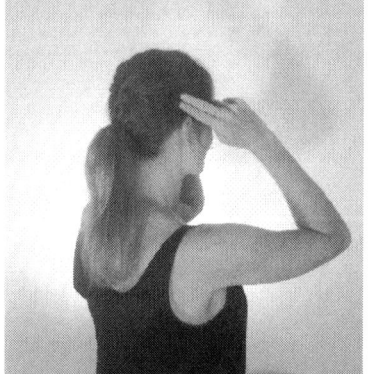

6. Place the fingers a little higher on the head from the previous point.

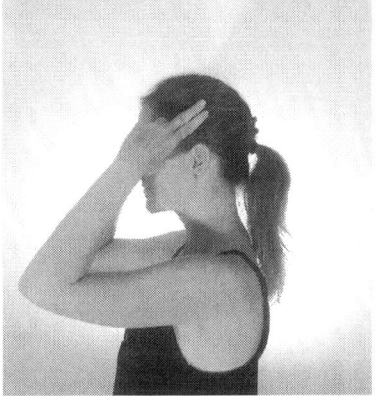

7. Place one set of fingers on the very top of the head.

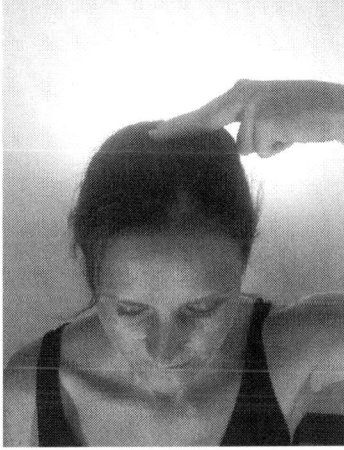

8. Place one set of fingers on the upper back portion of the head.

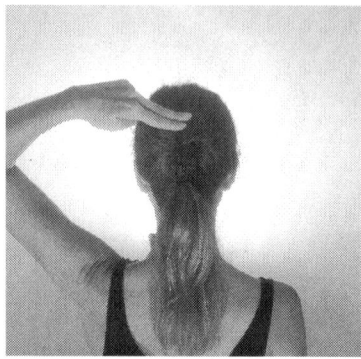

9. Place the fingers directly at the back of the head.

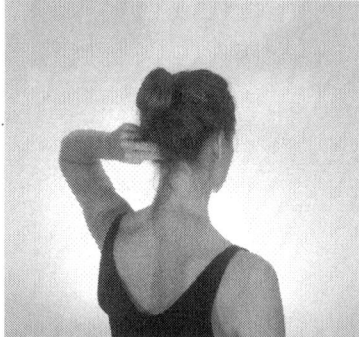

10. Place both sets of fingers on the back and sides of the head, well behind the ears and on the bone of the skull.

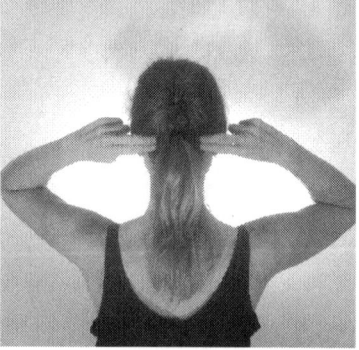

11. Place the fingers lower and into the occipital depressions off the bone and underneath the skull. Slightly lower then point 10.

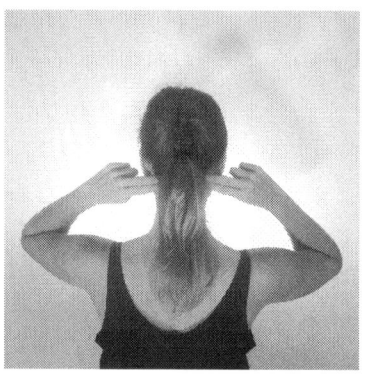 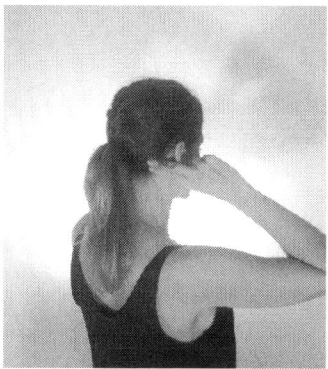

12. Finally, place one set of fingers just under the skull at the back of the head. A little lower then point 9.

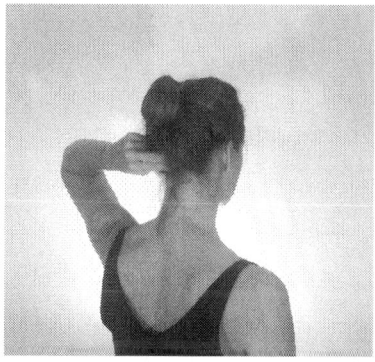

Giving Treatments to Another

Similar to doing self treatment, find a place where you will not be interrupted or distracted for 15 minutes. The person receiving treatment can sit in a comfortable chair—ideally a chair without a head support so that the person giving treatment can easily access the back of the head. It is best if the person giving treatment comes to stand just behind the person receiving it, so that the arms can easily access the head in a relaxed fashion.

If you have a massage table, or if the person receiving treatment would like to lie down on their back, then this is also an option. For the person giving treatment, make sure that you don't place your body into positions which create strain and tension. If the person receiving treatment is lying down, then in order to access the points on the back of the head, gently lift the head up so you can place your palms under the head, then come to rest your hands back down onto the table, pillow or floor. Adjust the hands slightly under the back of the head so as to access the points on the back of the head with the first and second fingers.

So the same fundamentals apply; just a light, gentle pressure of the fingers on the head, feel the warmth between the fingers and the head, and hold each point for about 45 seconds to 1 minute. Encourage the person receiving treatment to close the eyes.

1. Place the fingers on the first point on the front of the forehead.

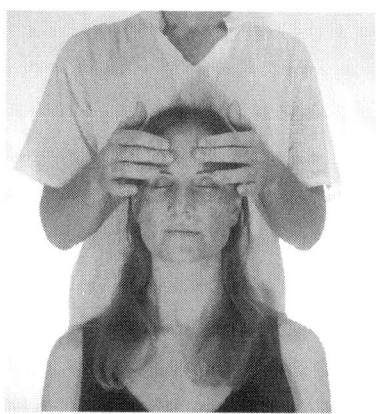

2. Place the fingers just behind the temples.

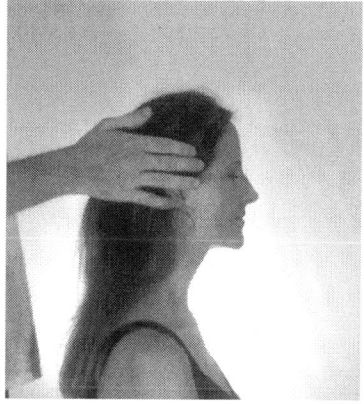

3. Place the fingers on either side of the jaw.

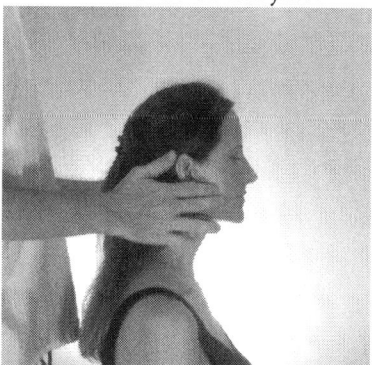

4. Place the fingers on the hairline directly above the eyes.

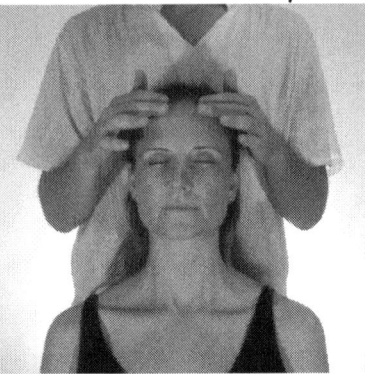

5. Place one set of fingers on the very top of the head.

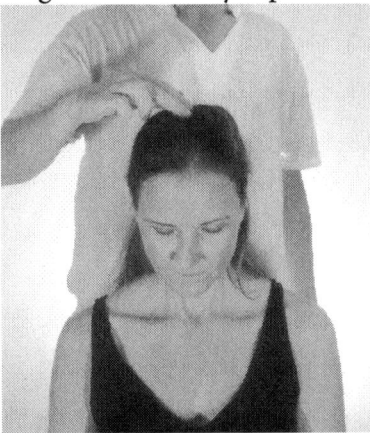

6. Place the fingers just above the ears.

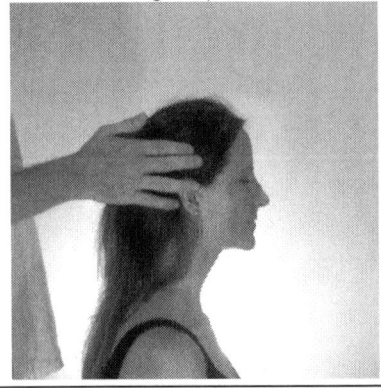 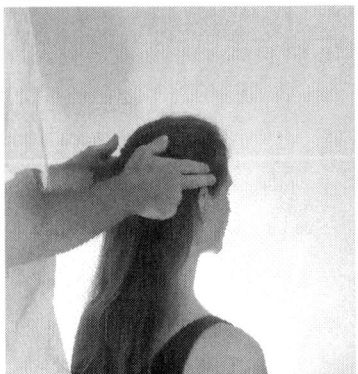

7. Place the fingers a little higher on the head from the previous point.

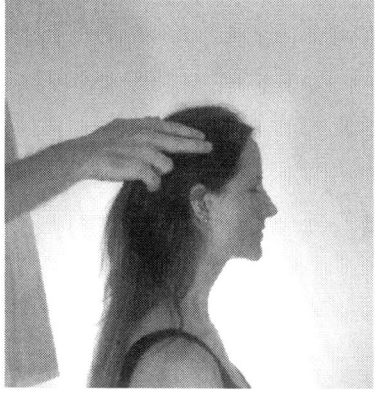 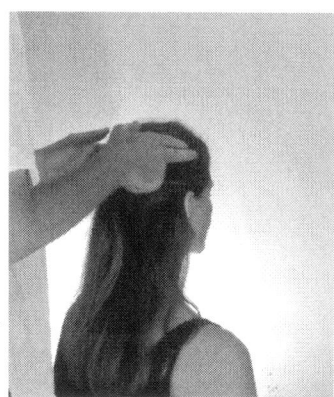

8. Place one set of fingers on the upper back portion of the head.

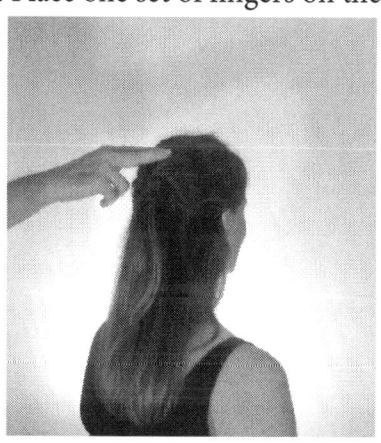 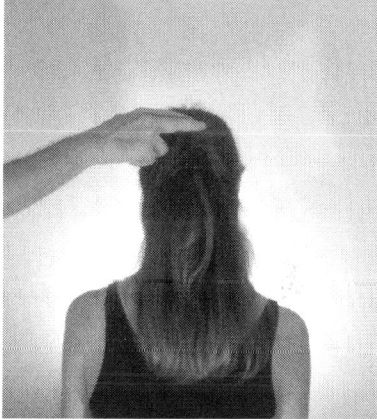

9. Place the fingers directly at the back of the head, on the bone.

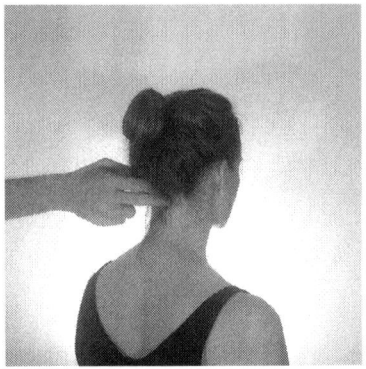

10. Place both sets of fingers on the back and sides of the head, well behind the ears on the bone.

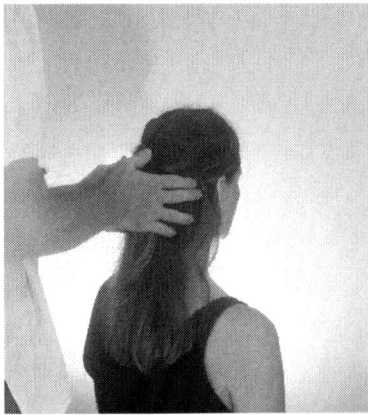

11. Place the fingers lower and into the occipital depressions , off the bone and underneath the skull.

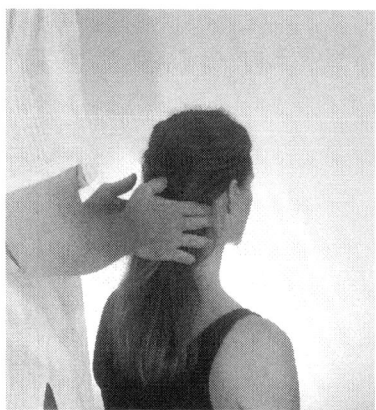

12. Finally, place one set of fingers just off the bone and under the skull at the back of the head.

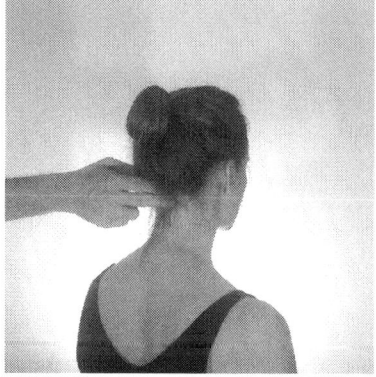

How Often to Practice?

This practice can be done on yourself or on somebody else at anytime, and as many times as you feel that benefits are gained from it. The whole process should take no longer than 10 minutes, and can potentially be done in only 5 minutes. If you don't have even that much time available, you can do just 3 or 4 points, and that may be enough for you to get a boost and rebalance your system. The most potent points I have found are:

Number 1 – GB 14 – on the front of the forehead
Number 6 – GB8 – just above the ears on the side of the head, and **Number 7** – DU 20 – on the very top of the head

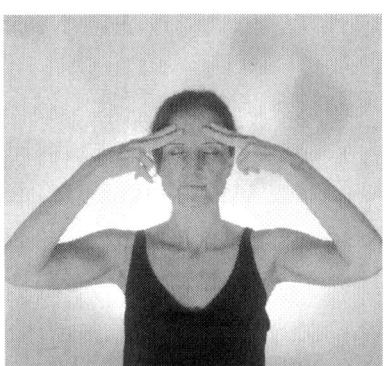 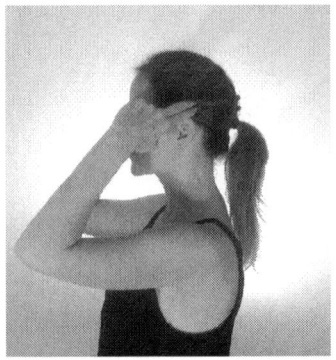

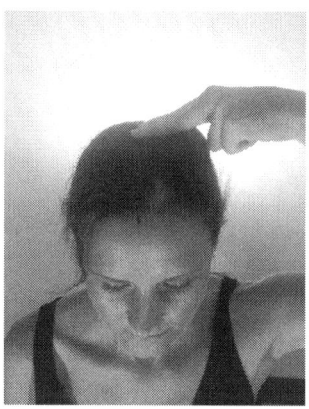

In my clinical acupuncture practice, I often used some of these points after I had given someone acupuncture. Sometimes treatments like acupuncture or massage can leave people feeling a bit groggy and vague, and I have found that if you use a few of these points after a treatment it quickly helps to reestablish the system and clear any grogginess. This can also be helpful to those people who find it hard to wake up, or who often feel groggy and vague for some time after waking. A few of these points will bring their system online a lot quicker.

If you often get headaches then I would suggest practicing this technique daily to see if it prevents headaches from arising. This technique would work best just before or at the initial onset stages of a headache, to help relieve any pain and dissipate any excess or stagnant energy in the head. Once the headache has taken hold this technique may provide some relief from the pain, but it is unlikely to clear it completely. However, it is worth experimenting with, because anything is possible. One thing to be aware of, though, is if the headache is stemming from tight muscles in the shoulders and neck, then it may be worth getting somebody else to give you a treatment so that you are not aggravating the tight muscles in the shoulders. This brings us into the subject of headaches, so let's talk about this in more detail.

Will This Help Me With Headaches?

The short answer to this is, yes, for most people. There are many causes to headaches, therefore there is not one particular treatment type that will cure all headaches. If you can identify what type of headache it is and what is causing it, you are well on your way to preventing headaches from reoccurring. Prevention is the best cure for headaches, because once they have taken hold they are often hard to clear without resorting to painkillers and/or locking yourself up in a dark room to sleep it off.

The most common causes of headaches are:

1. Muscle Tightness in the Neck and Shoulders

If a headache has taken hold and you are in a lot of pain and discomfort, then treatment suggestions would be to seek treatment from an osteopath, acupuncturist or good remedial massage therapist to bring the muscles out of their stressed state. If that is not an option for you in that moment, then taking painkillers and sleeping it off can help initially to clear the pain. For those who prefer a natural option, white willow bark is a natural anti-inflammatory that can act as an effective painkiller. It has similar properties to aspirin, so for those who have negative reactions to aspirin, it is best avoided. Once the initial headache pain has cleared, it is time to look at ways to avoid its return.

Once the muscles have eased off via treatment or some good quality sleep, it's your job to find a way to keep the muscles from tensing up again. This is really your job, as no one can really do this for you. If you get regular and consistent headaches from tight muscles in the neck and shoulders, even after regular treatments with massage therapists and other practitioners, then you need to work at changing your muscle movement patterns. The reason the tension and headaches keep reoccurring is because the movement behaviors of the muscles aren't working efficiently. If the muscles don't reorganize into a more efficient way of moving, then they will keep returning to the old patterns, which are causing the stress and the tension. Changing the behavior patterns of your movements can be done through movement style training that incorporates increased body awareness. The best method out there by far is the Feldenkrais method. There are group classes that one can attend, or one can see a trained Feldenkrais practitioner to get one-on-one treatments to help you reorganize your movement patterns. Feldenkrais classes are very gentle, and suitable for all levels. You can search for Feldenkrais classes in your area via the Internet.

The next suggestion would be gentle forms of yoga with an emphasis on building body awareness. Things like dance, or any form of movement training that emphasizes an increase in your body awareness, will help in changing the patterns of the body's movement behavior. What doesn't really help is slamming yourself at a gym, or running flat out on a treadmill while watching TV or reading a magazine. Most of the time, these activates and these approaches only increase the imbalances in the body because it reemphasizes poor movement behavior. Reorganizing movement behaviors generally involves slowing things down and placing our full attention on the movement itself. This gives the nervous system time to reorganize itself into more efficient ways of moving. And after any exercise or movement class, it is necessary to rest by lying flat out on the floor, or on a firm surface, for about 5 minutes with a relaxed body. This simply allows the body time to integrate the information of the movements, and again, gives the nervous system time to reorganize itself.

2. Stagnation of Energy

This is one of the main contributors to tight muscles in the neck and shoulders. The energy stagnation refers to the inability of the body to distribute energy smoothly throughout the body and to the brain. The feeling is of a foggy head, lots of sighing and a lack of the ability to concentrate. If left untreated it often leads people to become easily frustrated, and gives rise to a headache sensation behind the eyes. If you sit in the same chair for hours at a time, you can pretty much be sure that your body's energy is stagnating. The body is simply not designed to sit for long periods of time (generally, no more than 4 hours a day). The easiest treatment for this is to simply go for regular walks. If your job requires you to sit at a desk, don't despair—there are a few things you can do to avoid or reduce stagnation. Every 45 – 60 minutes, get up from your desk and go and do something else that requires you to move differently (e.g. stand, walk, look for things, prepare food, etc.). At your lunch break, after you've eaten (it is best to eat sitting down) go for a walk around the block. After work, go for at least a 30 minute walk. Keep the energy flowing and the body happy by moving the body's energy around. Again, you don't have to slam yourself at a gym or anything like that; a brisk walk for at least 30 minutes most days will often be enough.

3. Too Much Heat in the Body and Head

This is a Chinese medicine style description, as they often refer to conditions as being caused by imbalances of cold, hot, damp, dry and so on. In this case, heat in the body and head refers to a state when too much heat is trapped inside the body. Things like drinking too much coffee, smoking, drinking alcohol, and eating meat and sugary foods tend to load the liver up with toxins, leading to heat being produced in the liver. After some time, the heat tends to move upwards and accumulate in the head. Red eyes, red face, loud voice and a tendency to be easily frustrated or irritated are all signs that you may have too much heat inside your body and your head. It is also referred to as having too much yang energy. It can be cooled by drinking water and eating cool foods like salads and yoghurt, but foods tend to take a while (days, weeks or sometimes months depending on how toxic the liver is) to have any effect. If you want some immediate relief from a hot head style headache, then things like acupuncture, foot massages, diving into a pool or ocean, having cold showers, and the technique outlined in this book will all help to clear some of the heat and provide some pain relief more immediately. For ongoing treatment its best to avoid things that produce the toxic effect in the liver, like those things mentioned previously. Also, it is best to engage in activates that support the more gentle and nurturing side of your nature like resting, gentle yoga, meditation, reading books, eating nourishing foods and generally slowing things down, as these things don't tend to generate an excess of heat (yang).

4. Dehydration

Another common cause is dehydration. Dehydration headaches have their own unique type of feeling about them, usually felt across the front of the forehead. There is also a distinct lack of the ability to concentrate, and the mouth and lips are often dry. The best treatment is to drink more water! It is best not to drink ice cold or chilled water, as cold water taxes your body's energy, and it doesn't absorb quickly because the body has to heat it up to 38 degrees Celsius before it can absorb. It is best to drink it at room temperature, or even a little warm. Also look into rehydration formula drinks to get a hydration boost. For serious cases of dehydration, get to a hospital, as it can be life-threatening.

Working on Particular Issue or Stress

This practice is focused on clearing a specific stress from a past experience or an anxiety regarding the future. The following description is in the context of clearing stress for another person, however we can apply the exact same steps outlined and treat ourselves also.

For this treatment, we will use just 3 main power points. They are:

Number 1 – GB 14 – on the front of the forehead
Number 6 – GB8 – just above the ears on the side of the head, and
Number 7 – DU 20 – on the very top of the head

1. **Ask the person we are working with to bring a particular issue of stress to the mind.** Get them to say it out loud as it makes it more present and clear in the mind, e.g. "Last week my boyfriend broke up with me", "I have a very important presentation to make next week and I feel terrified", "Every time I think about . . . I feel anxious".

2. **Soon after we have brought the issue of stress it is a good idea to get a reference point as to how stressful the issue is.** Having a reference point will allow us to see how effective the treatment is. Now, let's get an idea as to how stressful this issue is using a scale from 1-10. Ask them, "On a scale of 1-10, 10 being maximum stress, when you think about this issue, what would it be?"

3. For the person who is giving, **come to gently place your first and second finger on the first point, GB14 – on the front of the forehead**. Ask the person receiving to gently close down their eyes. Now, get them to describe the stressful issue a little more by asking some simple questions about the event. Eg. When this happened, or will happen, what day was it? What time was or is it? Who was or is going to be there? We do this because we want to stress to be present while we use these points.

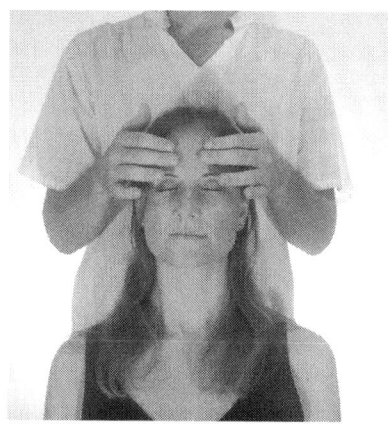

4. After 1-2 minutes. **Change our hand position and bring our first and second fingers to GB8 – just above the ears on the side of the head.** We can continue to speak a little more on the stressful subject, however it is not necessary. If the person receiving becomes quiet and silent – let them be silent, and just focus on offering your energy through your fingers.

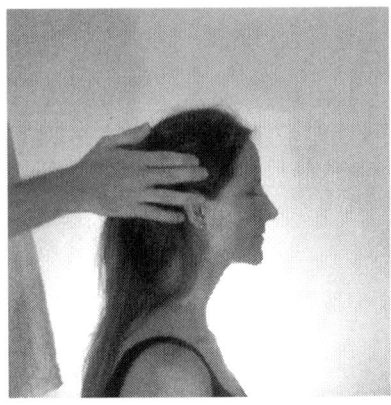

5. After 1-2 minutes, change our hand position and bring one set of fingers to the very top of the head at DU 20 – top of the head. Allow yourself and encourage the person receiving to become quiet and focus on some conscious breathing to help them let go and relax. Say something like, "Now, take a deep breath in... .and exhale... good."

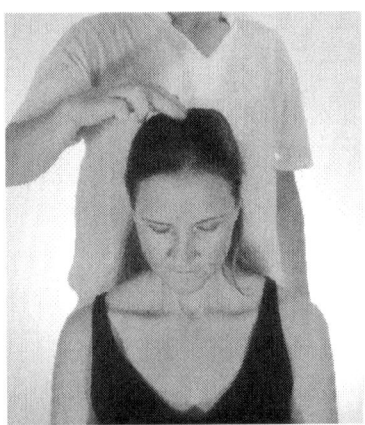

6. After 1-2 minutes, **as a nice way to finish come back to place your first and second fingers on the first main point GB14 – on the front of the forehead.** Now ask the person receiving if they can visualize the best possible scenario of the stressful event. You could also suggest visualizing the people involved in the event

looking at peace, happy, joyful and content. Then get them to visualize themselves at peace, happy, joyful and content.

7. After one minute release your hands and ask them to gently open their eyes when they are ready. Give the receiver a cup of water and take a moment for them to come back to the world.

8. Feel free to ask the receiver what the stress level is now when they think of the stressful event on the scale from 1-10 with 10 being the maximum stress. In most cases it will be down to around 1 or 2. If not, that is ok, if we have moved them just one or two points that can be enough. Often it takes time for people to re-organize into the new way of being with the stress. Therefore, whatever their response, take note and continue to offer support and comfort. Know that your compassionate efforts, energy and attention has reduced their stress whether they are aware of it or not.

Final Words

So there you have it, a simple and easy 12 point cranial relaxation technique to help you to calm the mind, nourish the eyes and balance out the nervous system in less than 10 minutes.

You now have a very powerful and simple healing technique that you can use on yourself and use it to help and support others. There are no negative side affects from this treatment.

Please feel free to practice this technique as much as you like. After you have practiced it on yourself, be sure to treat others with it. Also, feel free to show others the technique so they can do it for themselves. The more people who can practice simple energetic techniques such as the one in this book, the higher the potential for a calmer and more balanced world in which to live. When we are in a calm and balanced state, no ill-will or harmful actions can arise from within.

~ May All Beings Be Peaceful ~

*"Peace is the result of retraining your mind
to process life as it is, rather then as
you think it should be."*

~ Dr Wayne Dyer

Sign up for the author's New Releases mailing list
and get a free copy of *The Yin & Yang Lifestyle Guide*

Click here to get started:
www.michaelhetherington.com.au/freebook

Other Books By This Author

The Art of Self Muscle Testing
Learn how to access the human energy field for information

The Art of Self Adjusting
Learn how to stretch and make adjustments to the spine

EFT Through the Chakras
Work with EFT to clear the Chakras one by one

The Complete Book of Oriental Yoga
A journey into the 5 elements and yoga for the seasons

How to Do Restorative Yoga
Learn the art of a gentle yoga practice for deep relaxation

Increasing Internal Energy
Building energy from within to enhance daily life and strengthen
our yoga practice

Printed in Great Britain
by Amazon